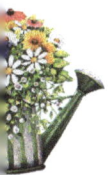

How to Step Out of Grief and Bloom: A Practical Guide

Stay engaged in the fight against grief. With the help of God, you will win!

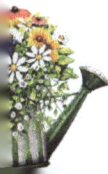

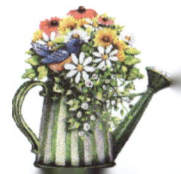

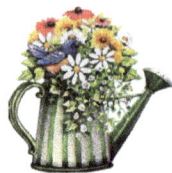

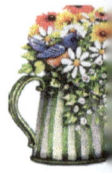

How to Step Out of Grief and Bloom: A Practical Guide
By
Diana Rowe

In this book, you will gain insights that will help you on your journey to overcome grief. You will learn about the stages of grief, self-care while grieving, your need for emotional support, facing grief, creating moments while grieving, processing depression while grieving, recognizing complicated grief, patience and forgiveness, and new perspective for your new normal.

Get your copy of the companion grief journal today.

Other Books by Diana Rowe:
Journal: How to Step Out of Grief and Bloom
Born to Die in My Place: A Timeless Story - Book 1
Born to Die in My Place: A Story of Unconditional Love - Book 2
An Invitation to the Sanctuary
An Invitation to the Sanctuary Lesson Planning Help for Teachers

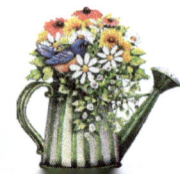

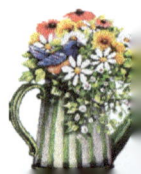

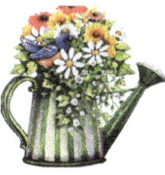

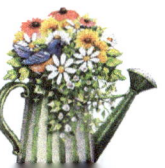

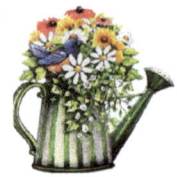

Table of Contents

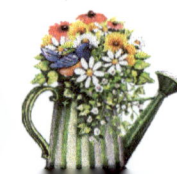

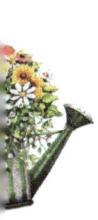
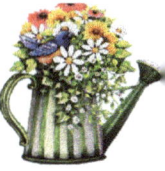

Dedication

This practical guide is dedicated to the many people who want to understand how to grieve in a healthy way.

I pray that God will guide your hearts and minds and strengthen you each day. And grant you the desire to live for His glory while being a blessing to others along the way.

Your friend on the journey,

Diana

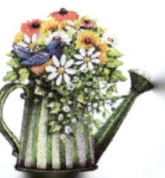

Lisa's story:

My name is Lisa. I remember my husband bringing me flowers every Friday. He would hide it behind his back and say, "guess what?" Of course, I would always say, "chocolate?" But he would say, "No, it is something as beautiful as you."

The week before he died, he surprised me with chocolate and a plant. I looked at him with a smile. Then we hugged. I asked him why he changed from flowers to a plant. He told me that he wanted to change things up and give me something that would last a little longer than the flowers. I really appreciated this plant, but I did not believe I had a green thumb. I loved my plant and watered it and placed it by the kitchen window for sunlight.

My husband was not feeling well that Tuesday morning, but he decided to go to work anyway. I didn't think anything of it. I gave him a couple of aspirins with his usual breakfast of oatmeal with berries, one hard-boiled egg and one slice of toasted whole wheat bread. I had a good day at work and came home to make dinner before my husband got home, except he didn't. That phone call, that ugly heart-stopping phone call; the call where nothing made sense and I was sure the hospital had the wrong name and number. I could not believe he was gone. How is this even possible. I was making his favorite foods; his birthday was coming up next Thursday. This is a very bad joke, or so I thought.

I must figure out how to fully inform myself that this was my life now. Other people told me they were sorry. I heard them and I politely said, "thank you." But I still did not inform me yet. I wanted to wait for the right time. I attended church that weekend as we often did but felt overwhelmed. As for that plant, I honestly thought the plant was dead, but I kept adding water and putting it closer towards the sunlight; after a while, I totally ignored it. I hated the plant but felt guilty to throw it away.

For weeks my relatives and friends came with food and encouraging words. I heard all of it and once again I politely said, "thank you." I was grateful but my heart would

6

not allow the words to penetrate to evoke any real emotion. I received lots of hugs from everyone who came by the house, and I listened as they shared how they will miss him and how their hearts break for me. My thoughts were racing, and I wished that my heart could break, at least I would know that it is still there.

Months after the funeral, I cried a lot. I found a few things in the album that made me smile for the first time, but I caught myself smiling and quickly stopped. It was as if I was breaking a law or something. It didn't feel right for me to be smiling. I finally got the courage to reach out to my best friend and told her what was happening to me and how I was hiding everything. She encouraged me to seek help and work through my feelings. That was good advice. I sought help but my friend was kind enough to provide me with some additional resources that saved me time and money.

I am so grateful for this practical guidebook. I learned about the stages of grief I was experiencing, and I am using the companion journal every day. I cannot tell you how much I learned and how the information is helping me right now. I had no idea that what I was going through was normal or that grief had stages. I appreciate that you as the author also shared personal stories of your grief and losses and can truly identify with those of us who are grieving.

I absolutely love the companion journal. This journal is unique and perfectly outlines everything I need to keep me on track with achievable realistic prompts when I didn't know where to begin. I love all the ideas and pictures in the journal. I really appreciate that you took the time to create a special journal for people like me who are grieving. Thank you for thinking about us. I am learning how to stop and pay attention to myself and others instead of just walking around in a maze. Example: While making a sandwich one afternoon, I saw something beautiful from the corner of my eye. Can you guess? It was the plant that my late husband gave me. It started to blossom! There was one tiny bud that was halfway open and another that was

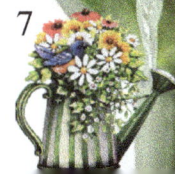

fully opened. My heart was flooded with joy. I started to see again, hear the birds, smell the fragrances around me. You would think this was the first time in my whole life that I saw a flowering plant. It's as if I was locked up in my grief and now, like the plant, I can finally blossom. This is what the title of the book suggests. My life can go on just like the plant.

I was so excited I called everyone I know, "my plant is blooming, my plant is blooming" was all I could say. My family members were all happy to hear me laugh; I also heard myself laugh and based on what I learned, I felt it was alright.

I will continue to use these resources and I am now helping others who are grieving to bloom. Thank you so much for allowing me to share my testimony,

Lisa.

Reply from the author, Diana Rowe

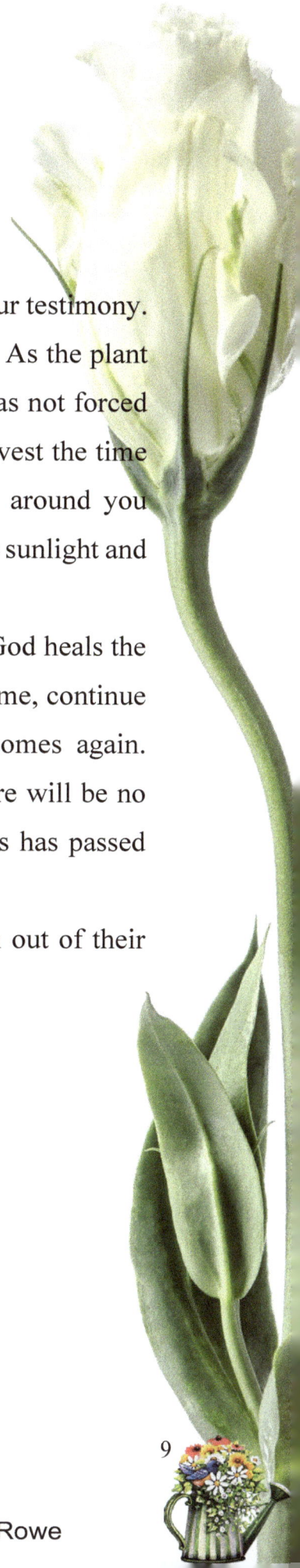

Hi Lisa,

My condolences to you. Thank you for being brave enough to share your testimony. I believe that God allowed this plant to be an illustration for your life. As the plant received all that it needed (water and sunlight), it knew no haste; it was not forced in any way it simply bloomed at the right time. God wanted you to invest the time and patience in yourself and to nurture yourself with the resources around you including time spent in prayer and devotion with Him. All these are like sunlight and water to the soul that helped you to bloom.

The same God who helped you can help others bloom. It is true that "God heals the brokenhearted and binds up their wounds." Psalm 147:3. In the meantime, continue to hope in God because you will see your husband when Jesus comes again. Revelation 21:4 says, "God will wipe every tear from their eyes. There will be no more death or mourning or crying or pain, for the old order of things has passed away."

God be with you and every person out there who will learn to bloom out of their grief.

Diana

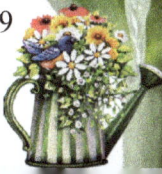

How to Step Out of Grief and Bloom: A Practical Guide By: Diana Rowe

Chapter 1: A Look at the Five Stages of Grief

Plants go through different stages before they get to maturity. Skipping certain stages may harm the plant and prevent it from growing. Most stages of plant growth include being covered under dark soil for a while; another stage includes pushing through that same dirt to get above. Get ready to push through the grief stages so you can bloom above that dark soil.

Grief is a complex cycle that comes with many stages and separate experiences that can keep us overwhelmed by the complexities of dealing with the loss of a significant relationship or situation. What may cause a person to experience grief? The death of a loved one, loss of a marriage that ended in divorce, loss of businesses and jobs, loss of significant relationships, loss of pets and so many things that people hold dear.

If you gather all the people in any given community, you will find that every group grieves differently based on several factors. An individual's culture can dictate the way he/she grieves. A person's religious background also has a tremendous impact on the way each person or family grieves. However, despite the differences, it is possible to move forward after dealing with a significant loss; there is hope that we can find peace and live a productive life.

Acceptance is usually the last stage of grief that we arrive at, and we can quickly move from acceptance to denial and return to denial all over again. Grief can take quite a while for us to process. Therefore, it is vital that we help ourselves through this process by understanding as much about grief as possible and being patient and forgiving with ourselves as we deal with the issues that are frequently associated with grieving and loss.

This course and the companion journal will help you to learn more about grief. Taking this course online or using the book shows that you are already aware of the responsibilities that you have toward yourself and your healing; this is a very positive step in the right direction and your strength and courage are admirable. When you are going through a difficult time with your grief, it can often be

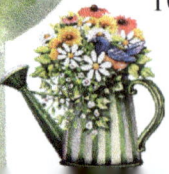

10

challenging to articulate and admit, let alone seek resources to help yourself. Congratulations on making it this far! You are stronger than you think!

According to the Kubler-Ross model (2009), there are five stages to the grief process. The five stages are Denial, Anger, Bargaining, Depression, and Acceptance. We will discuss these five stages of grief.

STAGE 1: DENIAL

Denial is the first stage of grief. When I heard the horrible news that my sister died, and at another time, that my father died, I was in denial. I could not accept it; I immediately told myself that it is not true. Have you ever been there? Then you understand what I am saying. Sadly, too many people are familiar with this heart-wrenching news. It is always hard to accept this reality, no matter how many times it shows up in our lives. So, what do we do? We hide that information in our denial mental file and run in the opposite direction in our minds.

God made our bodies with superb defense mechanisms to protect or quickly put distance between ourselves and trauma. Visualize a boulder coming at you. What would you do? You would move out of the way as quickly as possible and try to put something between you and the bolder to cushion the blow. However, if the boulder comes to our mind in the form of bad news, our brain tries to protect us from the shocking news. Denial almost gives us a minute away from absorbing the full intensity of this reality. In this sense, denial is like a shield of God's grace, not giving us more than we can bear at that moment. Unfortunately, we must face reality no matter how long we linger in a state of denial. But at least we can come out from denial one moment at a time.

Denial can be a very trying stage for you, other family members, friends, or strangers who are connected to the situation but maybe experiencing different stages of the grief cycle. When you are feeling like the news you just heard is too terrible to be accurate, and you check out of reality for a little while, do not be

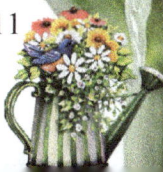

11

surprised if it is frustrating to others who are angry or depressed about the loss. It will not be easy for others to consistently reiterate the fact that yes, this is happening to us, and there is nothing that we can do to change this moment in time. They may not fully understand where you are in the cycle and why you might take so long to get to the stage they might be. Everyone may not remain in the same stage for the same length of time.

STAGE 2: ANGER

Anger is the second stage of grief. When things hurt us suddenly, it is not unusual for us to respond in anger. We do not want to drench in the feeling of helplessness amid our pain. It can be especially difficult if we know that there is someone still alive and malicious out there who is responsible for taking the life of our loved one. Feeling wounded unjustly or harmed can often signal our natural reflex towards anger. Whether we are angry at the subject of our loss for leaving, angry at others for how they are treating the loss, or mad at those who caused the loss, the end feeling is the same. Then there is rage toward Sovereign when we get angry at God who is sovereign, yet, He is nowhere around when this horrible enemy of death is stealing away someone precious to us. So, we rush to our default sovereign-blame, indirectly, of course: where is God? He must truly not be aware of what is happening because there is no way He could see this and not stop it instantly. Is there anything hidden from God? Keep on reading; you will come to a better understanding as you read.

Two of the most important questions from grieving hearts are: Why me? Why now? It is unfair and agitating to know that I am suffering for some unknown reason, or even for no reason whatsoever. But even worse, if we do know, and there is nothing we can do about it. A prime example is a disease or virus that attacks us without warning or preparation, and before we can understand

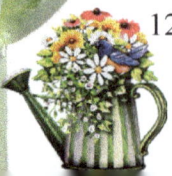

12

what is happening, our loved one is gone. How do we process this when we cannot see this invisible agent of death that snatches the life of those we love without any apology? One minute our family members go from a typical day with relatively decent health to battling for their life. Can someone explain this to our heart, please?

God created us with powerful minds that need to try to make sense of everything that happens to us, especially as we begin to emerge from under the shadow of the shock. Our minds want justice because the life of our loved one has value, and we crave the power to make any attempt to show that someone or something must be held accountable. After all, we do not believe that our loved ones should simply die in vain as if they are inanimate objects. So, we contend between cause and effect trying to make sense of what happened. In these moments, we are reminded in a very unambiguous way, that we are not in control of everything, and this situation is totally out of our hands. Things like death can be infuriating for many people when we are trying to maintain structure and control in our lives.

Although anger is negative in some instances, it can sometimes catapult us to taking decisive actions to regain our strength by looking beyond ourselves and looking to God to lift us up. I entered this arena of anger when I lost my eldest sister, whom we affectionately called, Precious. She was in the hospital and was to be discharged and return home, but instead, we heard the dreaded news that she died. I was in denial for a while. Months after the funeral, I was still angry, but mostly at Jesus, my God, my Savior, and the one who I also regard as my Friend since my early childhood. Yes, I love Jesus, and I know He loves me more than my human mind can comprehend. I had one question for Jesus, how could you allow my sister to die and not let me say goodbye? I thought we were friends. I continued to tell Jesus that I did not want to speak with Him, but if He wants to talk to me, I will try to listen. So, one morning after my usual prayer, thanking Him for waking me up, my heart was sad and disappointed with Jesus. At the same time, I missed Him,

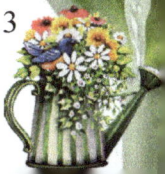

13

sharing with Him my every thought, before my anger strike. So, I said, Lord, I feel really hurt and sad today. Then I stopped talking, and the Lord directed my mind back to the last day I saw my sister alive: We arrived early at the airport so we could get something to eat and talk for a while. There were other relatives there too. But strangely, I spent the whole time at the airport with my head on my sister's shoulder as she held me and told me she loved me and to take care of myself until we meet again soon.

That memory revealed the grace and loving-kindness of Jesus. I said, Lord, you did give me one hour at the airport to say goodbye to my sister! You do care! The tears of relief came strolling down my face. My heart felt lighter, knowing that my Friend and Savior cared about the little things like goodbye, even though I did not realize it was that kind of goodbye. My anger dissipated, and I apologized to Jesus for being blinded by denial and pain that fueled my anger toward Him. I quickly asked Him for one of the usual hugs that He would give me. Yes, Jesus gives hugs. We sat and hugged as I sobbed, knowing that Jesus cares and understands my human perplexities.

Even if He did not show me those moments, I know eventually I would run back to Him because the nature of our relationship allows me to feel what I am feeling while being honest with Him. I know Jesus does not love me any less because I wonder why, or because I get angry. He patiently waits for me to come to a place of reasoning, knowing that He has no desire to cause me pain or hurt. His heart breaks to see me hurt. He gets no pleasure from seeing me in my pain. He truly is a God of love and compassion. Did Jesus give you a beautiful moment with your loved one, but your grief blocked it out? It does not matter how long ago; it is still essential.

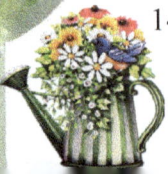

14

STAGE 3: BARGAINING

Bargaining is the third stage of grief. Negotiation occurs when we allow the knowledge about the loss to sink into our minds for a few moments. Because the pain reaches the very depth of our soul, we often feel we will do anything to reverse the adverse effects of the situation. We will make promises we cannot keep and even offer to change our attitude and be different in exchange for a favorable outcome. We will also bargain with God and tell Him that we will be better if He will just have mercy and take away this nightmare, just this one time. Our promises to God do not always change the result of our loss. Sometimes, we pray fervently before losing our loved ones and seek every specialist to look at their case. When we place our faith and hope in God who knows all things, we do not always understand God's love in allowing us to experience loss. It is difficult to comprehend God's love, allowing loss. We are not always prepared to see a loss in God-centered love.

When we are swept up in grief, we often feel like we would do anything possible to make the bad feelings that we are having disappear. Truthfully, most of the time loss that inspires grief is irreversible. Sure, we may grieve the loss of a friendship or relationship that could eventually repair if both parties are mature enough, but a lot of the times when we grieve, it is because of events beyond our control that we cannot reverse.

Bargaining with God was my second phase. So, the stages of grief do not necessarily follow a linear order. Different individuals can experience each step in a different sequence and may return to a previous phase. After learning of my sister's death, in and out of shock, I asked God if He could let me trade places with my sister. I felt that she deserved to live because she had two small children who needed their mother. My bargaining was clearly outside of God's providence. He had the big picture of our lives from the end to the beginning, and from the beginning to the end. I could only see my pain and loss.

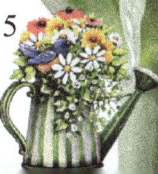

When we are grieving a death, for example, it is impossible to reverse the effects; and this knowledge can cause us to get trapped in the grim side of life for a long time, as the level of grief gets deeper and deeper; this is a natural place to be, though not forever. It is part of grieving, a course that the human body goes through to find equilibrium again with a new normal.

STAGE 4: DEPRESSION

Depression is the fourth stage of grief and often the most long-lasting and common stage. Grief can cause us to sink into the dark valley of depression; the problem is that many people get comfortable and can involuntarily stay for too long. This frozen state of existence is unhealthy for the body, mind, and spirit and will surely prevent us from seeing that our lives have worth that deserves dignity and quality.

Hence, depression is difficult to move through because we do not feel like moving at all. Most of the time, depression leaves us sluggish and unmotivated (Zhang & Yen, 2015). We would rather lie in bed and feel dreadful than get up and do the things that are expected of us. And sometimes that is alright. It can be what we need to take a break from the responsibilities of our everyday lives and begin to mentally and emotionally process our loss.

However, it can be a slippery slope. Sure, we can justify being depressed for a week or two after a shocking loss, but if that depression persists for too long, it can become a chronic state that we will discuss in a later section. Chronic depression can all but destroy our lives and the stability that we struggle to build, and if we allow ourselves to reside in this dangerous emotional state, it can have lasting consequences (Mahali, Beshai, Feeney, & Mishra, 2020).

Nevertheless, while we are grieving, the depression stage does not always throw us for a loop. We can be depressed healthily and allow ourselves to process the difficult emotions that are plaguing us. If we allow ourselves to move

16

successfully through the individual stages of grief to a place of acceptance, then we will not have to worry about depression impacting us immediately. Because this stage of grief can be so all-encompassing, we will discuss it more in-depth later in this course.

STAGE 5: ACCEPTANCE

The final stage of grief is acceptance. Acceptance can be something that we need to work very hard for, especially when struggling through the other four stages of grief. It may take quite a few cycles before we reach a permanent state of acceptance. Many people might think that the sequence of grief is an easy list that we all experience one by one in perfect order until we reach the end, but unfortunately, that is not the case. Sometimes people cannot reach acceptance permanently until the cycles of grief have been experienced several times over, at times, very out of order. You can never predict how you will respond and how many times you can find yourself in a specific stage while grieving. Some may argue that it is impossible to reach permanent acceptance. But, you can, not because you rush to get there on your own, but because God can help you do so in a way that works for you.

Remember, as individuals, we experience life in different ways, and that includes our emotional turmoil. The grief process knows no haste or specific date from beginning to end. Moving forward takes your daily life and breaks it down into little moments of attainable, realistic steps. Grieving is not a competition; that is why the companion journal allows you to personalize your pace to achieve daily success towards acceptance and beyond.

Acceptance is something that eluded me after the loss of my father. I knew that he had died. I was at the funeral. I viewed him lying so still in his favorite suit. I touched his cold cheeks and reminisced of the many hours we talked, and his infectious laughter would fill the room. He looked just the way he did when taking a nap at home, so peaceful. I tried to cry but smiled instead.

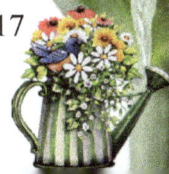

17

I did all that I could do to focus on helping anyone else who needed some cheering up. After a few days, I went back to work and immersed myself in my work. A year went by, and I encouraged my family members, especially my brother, who shared the same birthday with dad. I prayed even more than before. I drew closer to God with gratitude that I had a heavenly Father that will be with me always. In the second year (on the anniversary of dad's death), I got home from work with an unshakable burden. I felt like a cup about to overflow but not sure why.

I went inside and ran to my room, threw myself across the bed, and cried for more than an hour; real loud pillow-blocking, heart pour-out cry. After that, I asked myself what just happened and how is it that I am crying so hard two years later, when I could not cry before. I spoke with a pastoral counselor, and he assured me that my experience was not unusual. He further stated that I was finally accepting my father's death and allowing myself to feel the loss on a deeply emotional level, even though I understood the loss mentally. So, it was time; and my body could not hold everything anymore; I had to let it out.

Interestingly, I felt refreshed and at peace. I did not feel any anger or sadness. Although I was up and about doing my routine, I did not realize that two years later I would still be grieving. I had friends who told me that after a few months to a year, I should be over it. So, I certainly did not know that it would take two years for me to accept my father's death finally. I am glad I did. I had no idea that the passing of time did not mean that I accepted the loss. Thank God for His peace and for creating intelligent bodies that respond to trauma while patiently remembering to activate internal care by setting aside an unknown time for a good cry that promotes self-emptying healing.

When I reached acceptance, I felt the peace of God, not calmness without peace. But Godly peace within the mental-emotional ownership of suffering a loss.

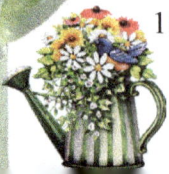

18

And allowing God to flush out my pain and give my heart rest assured me that He still has me and my healing in His hands. So, when I think of my late sister or dad, I feel grateful to have shared a part of my life with them. I thank God for giving me the grace and strength to continue to honor their memory with my life. Perhaps you are still struggling here. But you can ask God to help you, not to skip over the process, but to sustain you during the process without allowing grief to extract all of your hope. Moreover, there is nothing wrong if you have the occasional cherished memories, whether with tears or laughter. Removing the pain does not mean forgetting the person; you are merely choosing to remember in a healthy way that does not cause you to stress or deplete your resilience to thrive.

Thus, acceptance enables us to resolve the other pieces of the grief stages and organically embrace the fact that the loss happened. Arriving at peace will help us to move on from the crushing and seemingly insurmountable grief to continue living our lives to the best of our God-given abilities. Is this possible for you? Can you truly have peace? Yes, you can! Have you met the Prince of Peace? His name is Jesus. "For He (Jesus) Himself is our peace…" Ephesians 2:14. Jesus said, "Peace I leave with you, My very own peace I give to you; I do not give you the kind of peace that the world gives. So, do not let your heart be troubled or fearful." John 14:27. When you allow Jesus, the Prince of peace, to place His peace in your heart, you can be at peace with any situation, including the loss of a loved one. Ask Jesus to give you His peace right now. Believe that He will because He can; He loves you! Make a note in your journal about this request.

Use the grief journal to record the stages of grief that you are experiencing.

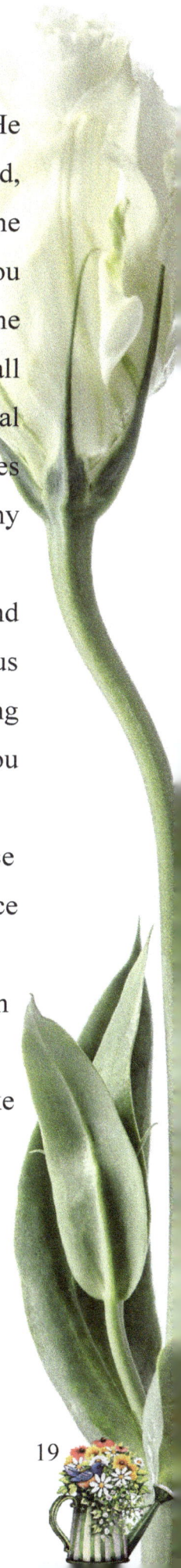

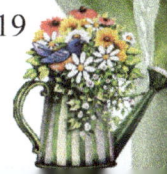

Chapter 2: Common Symptoms of Grief

When a plant is sick, it can show symptoms such as ringspot or leaf distortion. Plant owners often try to find the underlying cause and take the necessary course of action to help restore the plant. As you grieve, carefully examine your symptoms so that you can take actions that will not impede your progress to bloom.

Grief makes you curious, even anxious, to know why you're suffering. Grief can cause you to question everything when you are facing a loss you may not expect. Also, when you anticipate a loss due to prolonged illness or a fatal diagnosis, the experience is still painful. Thus, understanding the symptoms of grief can help you maneuver how you will respond to the people around you and how you will treat yourself during this time of significant loss.

These symptoms do not occur in any particular order:

1. SADNESS

Sadness is an everyday emotion that is familiar to all of us. However, when we experience a loss, this sadness is compounded with helplessness and confusion about what is happening. We can feel that our emotions are highjacked by some strange, unimaginable crime against our hearts and lives that zaps our mood and drag us to an unhappy place. Suddenly, we realize that all the power over our situation is not in our hands, and we hunger for a sense of familiarity. Nevertheless, as we go through the cycles of grief and use helpful resources, we can experience less sadness. Additionally, during this time of sorrow, you can pray and ask God to cheer your heart with a song, a Bible text, a pleasant memory, or even a kind response to someone else who is suffering a similar or other loss.

2. CRYING

One of the outlets that allow our bodies to escape some of our sadness is crying. Avoidance does not mean that we do not face or experience the grief that is infringing upon us; it means that our bodies are created to react to the sadness and

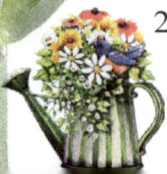

find a healthy, positive solution to let it out. Even though crying can be a short-term relief, it can really improve your mood. There is something therapeutic about crying when we lose a loved one. So, if you feel your eyes welling up with tears, go ahead and cry. This reminds your heart to simply let it out, let it all out, and this emptying of sadness through crying is healthy for you to do. Do not feel that you need to justify why you are crying. It's alright to cry. In the many cases of sadness brought on by painful or disappointing situations, we do cry. However, we must be vigilant to monitor our emotional sadness while we grieve, so we do not dive into the complexity of deep despair, which can lead to depression.

Crying, according to researchers, is helpful for our bodies. Our emotional tears are different from basal tears that help to moisten our eyes or reflex tears that are triggered by external irritants like onions. Emotional tears, however, contain multiple stress hormones and chemicals that help to ease our physical and emotional pain to promote wellness (Vingerhoets, 2013). God is so amazing in the way He created our tears to release a little help to cope in these times of grief. So, do not suppress your tears or ignore the role of crying during your grieving cycles.

3. DISBELIEF

Disbelief is another symptom of grief when we are facing the loss of loved ones. It is not unusual to have the same behavioral expectations immediately following the loss. When my friend, M.J., lost her twin sister, she was in denial for a long time. She watched the front door for days; she waited by the window to see if her sister would come walking up the path towards the house, but that did not happen. When she heard a key in the door, she ran with expectancy, only to be disappointed by the reality that her twin sister and best friend was not coming home. She described her feeling as one of numbness. I am sure many people can relate to those feelings throughout the grieving process.

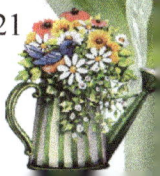

4. GUILT

Guilt is another symptom that can grip the heart and mind and leaves a person feeling frozen or stuck in place. It is easy to stay in the mindset of "what did I fail to do or what did I do that wasn't enough?" Also, "did I hurt this person in any way? What did I say in our last conversation that I didn't get to apologize for?" When it comes to guilt, the list has no end in sight. Death, and often divorce, cuts us off from the usual routine of interacting with our loved one; so, all the conversations are now taking place in our minds with no place to go. It is difficult for us as humans who are accustomed to continuity and coming to natural closures in our communication with others, or at least we get to decide that we will pick up where we left off in the conversation later. Therefore, death can seem like an abrupt intruder. We can all agree that we feel robbed by death.

How do I get beyond this feeling of intense guilt? How do I move forward on a journey toward healing? There will be more to come on this subject in a later section.

5. FEAR

Fear and anger are common symptoms of grief. These two emotions are closely related. When people are experiencing fear, it can manifest in outward or inward anger; and anger is often driven by fear of some kind. When we lose someone that we love, it is easy to develop feelings of bitterness. We may often shift the blame between ourselves and others for not doing more to save those we love. We may wreck our brain trying to rationalize whether our loved one is to blame in any of this. It is especially painful if the person decided that living is unbearable, and they would rather not live.

When a crisis occurs, we still hope for the best, and at times we have a method in mind for getting through to the other side. One moment you're enjoying a normal life with family and friends and the next, you are battling in the fight of your life.

How to Step Out of Grief and Bloom: A Practical Guide By: Diana Rowe

In times like these, you will do all that you can with the help of God to survive and thrive. Sometimes, that includes enlisting the skills of trained professionals to sort out the situation. We know that life has no guarantee, but it challenges us to be optimistic, even amid life's storms.

Are you feeling fearful after a loss? You are not alone, and your feeling is not uncommon. There are times when this fear can make you think that it is better not to expect any joy or happiness ever again because you will not be able to keep it; this is not a realistic picture to accept for your life. It is a temporary outlook that is born out of your pain, disappointment, and loss, and if not checked, can lead to anxiety. You do not want to live in a state of panic all the time or constantly worry about what will happen next. If you feel yourself staying in this space too often, you may need to seek a trained counselor who allows you to feel safe enough to share where you are emotionally without judging you for feeling that way. You can also seek God who is by your side; ask Him to remove the fear, and He will help you to cope and move into the joy that He has in store for you. "When I am afraid, I will put my trust in You/God." Psalm 56:3. God knows that we can be afraid at times, and He wants us to come to Him when that happens. God wants us to consciously and actively participate in the joys of this present moment.

God says, "Do not be anxious about anything, but in everything by prayer and supplication with thanksgiving tell Him your requests. And the peace of God, that surpasses all understanding, will guard your hearts and your mind in Christ Jesus." Philippians 4: 6-7. Anxiety and trust in God cannot exist in the same instant because anxiety shows distrust in God and puts the focus on self and our abilities to control what will happen next. But God is the only one who knows the future, and He can give you peace today and, in the future, as you begin to trust Him. He reigns over all the issues that confound you. He is God. The God of the universe loves you and wants you to be well.

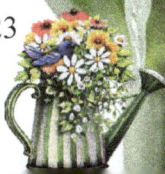

23

It is also important to remember that Jesus is our heavenly Counselor. He is more than able to cast out all your fears if you surrender them to Him. "When anxiety was great within me, your consolation brought me joy." Psalm 94:19. Remember that God does not give us the feeling of fearfulness or anxiety. In 2 Timothy 1:7, the Bible tells us that God does not give us fear; instead, He gives us power, love, and self-control. Hence, God will provide you with the power that provides the strength necessary to oppose and rebuke fear, which is rejecting the spirit of bondage, refusing to be a prisoner of fear. God will also give you love for who you are in Him. You can demonstrate this in your willingness to allow Him to help you to love yourself, which will enable you to be gentle and patient with yourself during your time of grief. The self-control here is God helping you to discipline your mind to accept your new normal and not allow yourself to accept defeat. Take control of your emotions and where you allow your thoughts and actions to focus; be intentional about what you will do in the present moment and do it. You can start by making a list. Get out your companion journal and make your list.

Fear and anxiety crush or weaken a person and can paralyze you and prevent you from even desiring to be happy or to go outside. Having God's love, power, and self-control is to receive a balanced new normal. You must execute the power and the self-control in love. Therefore, you can lovingly remind yourself that "I am not going to allow this loss to destroy me; memories, I will enjoy by laughing or crying. But I am going to live with God's love, power, and self-discipline; I am going to give that which is kind and uplifting to others and myself."

Chapter 3: Self-Care While Grieving

For a plant to bloom, the soil must be prepared. Consider your self-care like preparing the soil of your body, soul, and mind with the water, food, rest, and other activities that will help to nurture and eventually cause you to bloom.

Cultures around the world grieve in different ways; however, we all have something in common: sympathy and empathy. People demonstrate their compassion for others who are grieving through the giving of their time, talent, food, monetary donations, music, words of encouragement, doing errands, and more. Families, friends, and sometimes strangers will step up to help during times of loss.

Grief is something that we feel on a global level; thus, people all over the world must engage in self-care. Grieving is a life-changing cycle that affects every aspect of our lives. We don't see our daily needs the same way. When it is time to eat, we may not feel hungry. Our regular schedule to get out of bed and shower or make breakfast will look different. The motivation to clean up our surroundings and maintain our healthy habits can be lacking. Do you see why family, friends, neighbors, and community come out to help? The people around you do understand this, and they respond to the need by dropping off food and gifts or offer to help you around the house or if you need something done outside. Some people offer to listen quietly and allow the grieving person to talk; some may comb or style a person's hair just to help them to feel better; others may offer a word of encouragement, pray with, and for the person who is grieving.

Therefore, take note of the people around you who want to help, and do not be offended if they want to do something that you didn't think of or something that might seem personal to you. They are not trying to offend or hurt you; they just want to help you. When you lose a loved one, that is a substantial emotional and mental pain that affects the way you do life, but you don't always see yourself and how you might have deviated from what used to be your normal. The people around us will

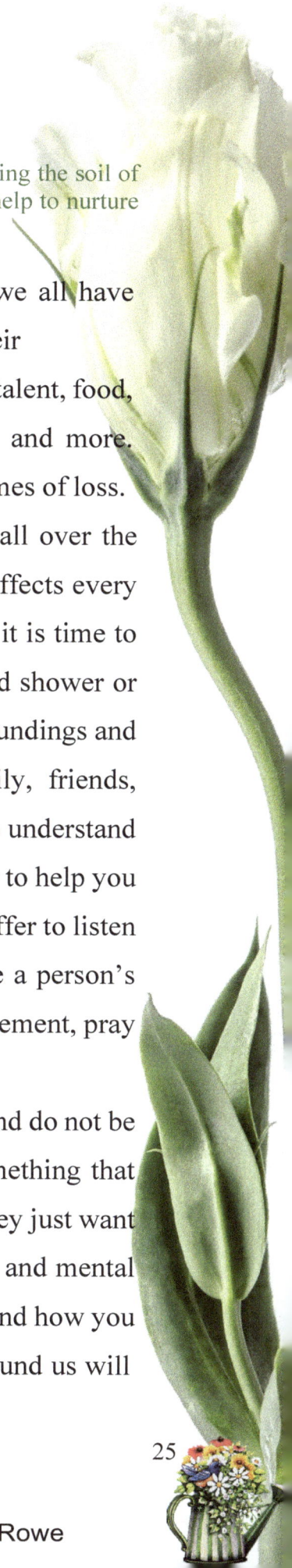

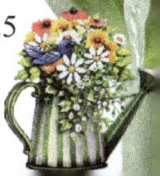

notice that we are having trouble caring for ourselves, and we do not need to feel shame; this is normal.

Allow people to help you. Accept the advice of family and friends who are interested in your well-being. If someone reminds you to eat, pause, and eat. If someone wants to prepare a meal for you, let them do it. It can help to inspire the attitude of care in your mind, especially as you may not be able to observe that you are falling into a state of disrepair.

CAUTION: Try to avoid extended grief that causes you to indulge in unhealthy habits. Seek professional help immediately or call a friend or family member and let them know what is happening. Quickly inform them that you need their help to find the right resources to help you. Do Not Be Ashamed to Ask For HELP. The last thing you want is to sink further and further into a pit of depression with no escape.

Self-care can seem unnecessary and overwhelming at times. Some people may even think it is selfish to take care of themselves after losing a loved one. Why? Because psychologically, they may feel unworthy to be here; others may think that they need to punish themselves or neglect themselves because there is nothing to live for anymore. This is not the correct mindset for any person who is grieving. You have a right to be here. God has kept you alive for a purpose known to Him. Cherish the fact that you are worth being alive. Your life matters!

It is time to make each day count even if you don't feel like it. See ideas in your journal. Your journal has sections for your daily list of things to do; it has a self-care list to remind you of what you need to do to care for yourself; it has encouragement and prayer and questions that will help to walk you through this journey of grief. There is a lot of benefit in the grief journal that was created especially for you. As you use your journal each day, you will get back into the routine of caring for yourself in a new way that is practical, meaningful, and very beneficial for you and those around you. Your health matters, you need to heal from emotional wounds.

Remember that God has given you His power to strengthen your resolve to take care of yourself. Besides, God, Himself, is invested in your care. He will take care of you; you are not alone.

In addition to the journal, you can ask a friend or family member to hold you accountable. It will ensure that (1) you are actively taking positive steps forward, and (2) you are challenging yourself to think about living by planning and interacting with others instead of retreating alone. A supportive network is critical to get through this. The little things like brushing your hair or washing your face will no longer seem overwhelming once you start to feel productive again. The fact that someone is holding you accountable and checking on you will increase the chances of getting things done. It worked very well for my friend, Judy. She had small children, and she needed the structure of the companion journal to help her with looking after herself so she could gain strength and confidence to be present for her children.

Reading a daily encouragement or prayer before getting out of bed is always a great practice to get you motivated for the day ahead. You can say something like, "Father in heaven, thank you for waking me up to spend another great day of giving to myself and giving to others in need." When you feel encouraged, you will purposefully try to make a list of the things that you need. For example, take a moment on Sunday to list things you need to do during the upcoming week. Just write as things come to mind. After making this list, you can add it to the calendar on your phone or other gadgets if possible. Make sure to add a time for your breakfast, lunch, and dinner. Oh yes, this is very important. Write a time for your morning devotion with God. Your spiritual health is crucial to your overall health. Spend a quiet moment with God in the morning just thanking Him for the ability to move and breathe and share your gifts and talents in ministry to others. If you feel yourself wavering throughout the day, just pause and pray. "Lord I need your strength; help me to finish this day strong."

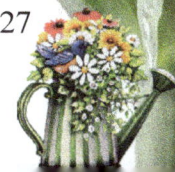

Remember, your basic needs are first and foremost, and if left neglected other things will most likely be left undone. It is not selfish to look after yourself first. Just apply the method used on airplanes; you must put the oxygen mask on yourself first so that you can help someone else.

Did you know that water can refresh you? Something as simple as a shower can help you to feel good about yourself. When we are clean and well-fed, it affects us mentally and physically. Ever wonder why babies are often more pleasant and playful after a bath and a bottle? O.K., so you're not a baby, but you get the idea. You are God's little son or daughter anyway.

According to researchers, cold showers can increase our oxygen intake and heart rate and make us more alert; it improves our circulation and lowers blood pressure, stimulates weight loss, and improve our overall health. Using cold water also helps people who suffer from anxiety and depression (Shevchuk, 2008). Hot showers release growth hormones to speed up the recovery of damaged cells in our bodies; the steam helps to detox the body as we sweat; and it helps to ease anxiety (Shevchuk, 2008). A shower is just one thing on the list for self-care, but do you see how beneficial it is for mental and physical health? Do not ignore the small stuff.

Do not under estimate the significance of self-care during times of grief. You must do everything in your power to recognize your obligation to yourself and others. You can overcome your grief; someone is waiting to hear your testimony. You are learning as you live through this difficult time; you are also teaching yourself and others who are looking on, that it is possible to bloom like a flower even after the storm. You are more resilient than you think. Do not allow your pain to enslave you or own you.

Chapter 4: Your Need of Emotional Support

Sometimes a plant gets damaged in the wind and needs external support to stand upright. Without this support, the plant may not rise to its full potential as it can remain bent and be cut off from the nutrients it needs to grow. Like a plant, the winds of life can damage us, and we need that extra emotional support from those around us while we grieve to help us to stand so that we can bloom.

It is not advisable to try to embark upon overcoming grief alone. Sometimes it can be almost impossible to do so. Grieving is a universal issue, but at the same time, the process looks different for each person. So, there is room for sympathy and empathy from those who may seem not to understand what we are going through.

When the going gets tough, a lot of times we tend to withdraw from family, friends, church, and other community engagements. It is not a good idea to isolate even though there are times when being alone for a moment can be beneficial to help us to examine ourselves and chart out some next steps. Nevertheless, we should not disregard the need for emotional support that our social structures and peer groups can provide. To do so can force our friends and family members to worry about us from afar. Is this what you want for your friends and family? I don't think so.

As much as we might feel that being alone can help us to heal, in truth, the support of other people is what we need during times of grief. Although it can seem complicated and unwanted, being around your community and being part of a group of people who genuinely care about you can help you to speed up the healing that you need during a time of loss. Not only that but allowing other people into your life can help you to get out of the house and into new situations where you're forced to face life and interact with others instead of being locked away with negative thoughts and your pain.

CAUTION: Grief can turn us into people we didn't know we could be. We can have extreme emotions and outbursts that we don't mean. We might lash out at others or take things the wrong way because we're feeling vulnerable and raw. So, it makes sense that we withdraw. It makes sense that we don't want to surround ourselves

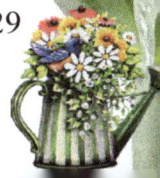

29

with those we might hurt or who might hurt us when none of us mean to hurt each other. The ironic thing about this is that without the support of others, the isolation we find comfort in can become permanent.

Did you know that most people find it difficult to ask for or accept help during times of grief? Sometimes people are afraid and decide to protect themselves from any situation that may cause indirect injure to their heart. No, there is nothing wrong with feeling that way. The grieving process brings all kinds of feelings and emotions that can make us feel vulnerable.

However, a lack of emotional support can push you further into isolation, and that can be dangerous for your progress to overcome grief. Don't settle into the mindset that no one cares or understands your pain. That is not true. People do care, and yes, they do understand. But if you are convinced that someone does not understand your grief, help them to understand by sharing how you feel and how they can best provide healthy and positive emotional support. You don't want your family and friends to think that you are somehow bitter, resentful, or punitive towards them because they are trying to be there for you.

Don't lose who you are; don't allow grief to re-brand your identity, negatively, especially after a death or divorce. Take your time to decide how you want to allow others inside your space without feeling that they are violating your need to isolate yourself. Just tell them what you need. Sometimes, you may only need a hug and reassurance that even though it feels impossible, things are going to turn out all right. "…With God, all things are possible." Matthew 19:26. Your support group will remind you that you will come out of this season of your life stronger than you believe. Perhaps you need silence; tell them and let them know that you are grateful that they take time out to care about you; just knowing that they are there makes all the difference, and it is very much appreciated.

How to Step Out of Grief and Bloom: A Practical Guide By: Diana Rowe

Do not push your support group away, even when they don't have the right words to express how they can help you. Grief is a deep and complicated process that can sometimes change our lives forever. So, if your emotional support group is having a hard time figuring out how to approach you, it's not because they don't care. Remember that they cannot read your mind or be inside of your feelings to have your real experience at that moment. So, help them to help you by sharing your needs and see how they will gladly do their best to assist—having this kind of support while grieving can be like a balm over painful emotional wounds.

Select your company wisely.

When you're forced to face life and react to external events, the stages of sorrow seem to go a little more smoothly, at least that's true if you keep good company. However, it's important not to make the mistake of surrounding yourself with people who will deplete you. For example, you don't want to have emotional support from people who are inconsiderate and selfish, who care more about themselves and petty problems than they care about being there for you. Be mindful when choosing who to spend your time with, because it's just as harmful to spend time with the wrong people as it is to avoid emotional support from others altogether.

Now that you know what type of individuals to avoid, here are some people that you can count on throughout times of need. Most of the time, these are people who will assist you and offer you the emotional support that you need to stay on a path of recovery. Family members and friends are excellent sources of emotional support. It can be helpful to remain in contact with other people who may be experiencing a loss or the same type of loss as you're experiencing but remember that these people are dealing with their own phases of despair and may not always be available to support you in the way that you need. Regardless, there's nothing quite like being close to people who are or have been through a similar tragedy.

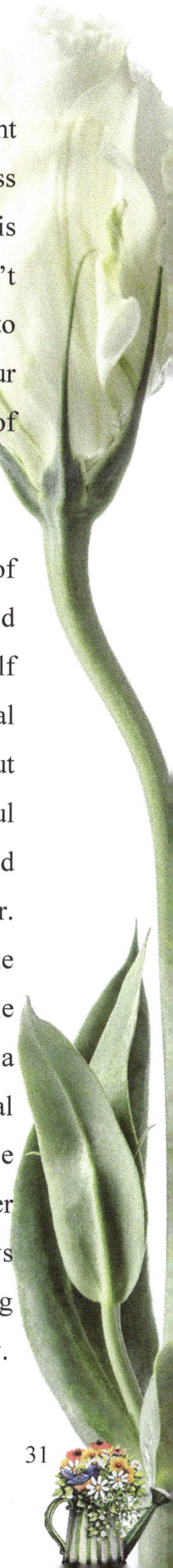

Being there for each other can be truly uplifting (if you do not pull each other into a deep dark emotional place every time you connect). Otherwise, it is a remarkable way to find validation in your emotions and make great friends who can genuinely understand how you feel in a manner that other people will not be able to. As 1 Corinthians 10:24 states, try to do what is good for others, not just what is good, for yourselves.

You can also find emotional support from your church family. Seeking comfort in God's guidance and through your church can be great for emotional support. Your church family will likely be there during times of need and utilizing these resources can be a great way to strengthen your faith and form bonds with like-minded people who want to help you move through the grieving process.

According to Romans 15:1, we who are strong should help to bear the burdens of those who are weak and not to please ourselves.

No matter where you find your emotional support (in a positive environment) what's important is that you hold on to it even when times prove to be difficult and challenging. Overcoming grief can be a considerable issue in your life, but with the right people, sharing the burden can make it that much easier for you to move on and begin healing. God can carry you through, and He can use other people to help you. Write the names of positive people in your grief journal.

Chapter 5: Facing Grief

A plant in the midst of a storm cannot pick up its roots and leave immediately; it has to face the storm. The great palm tree may bend and be tossed back and forth by the massive force of the wind, but the roots remain in place. You have the capacity to face your grief; your roots are deeper than you think. You can face your grief and survive to bloom in the days ahead.

Why is it vital for us to gain the courage to face our grief? Is it even possible to do this? Yes, it is possible to face grief. We cannot wait for all the pain to dissipate and then face our grief. We must be willing to consciously be in the here and the now. During this exact situation, Jodie, who lost her mother, did a simple surroundings check that was helpful: "stop for a moment and check the calendar." "Speak out loud so that you can hear yourself saying the name of the month, date, and time." "Look inside the room where you are and say out loud, I am here at this time, on this day, so that I can make a difference in this world." "I know I am grieving, but this is not the totality of my life." Speaking these words will remind you to actively engage in the process of facing grief while looking beyond the pain to see yourself as an essential contributor to your own life and the lives of others in society.

Some people say that grieving is all the love that we have for someone or something without being able to give it to them. Since it has nowhere to go, it stays in us and makes us sad. That is one way to look at grief and acknowledge that it is real. However, the reality is that love for people does not go away because we lose them, nor should it cause sadness. Instead, we can love many people who need someone to care about them. Sharing the love with others does not reduce or eliminate what we feel for those who died. We have the capacity to love during painful situations and even more after our pain while respecting the memory of those who died. This is also true for divorce.

CAUTION: Not facing grief creates a tedious process that harms the one who is grieving and the people around them. Grief is a normal experience, and we do not

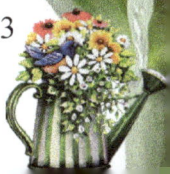

33

want to make it more difficult than it has to be. Consequently, it is best to face your grief without pretending that you're doing fine. Those who love you do not expect you to tell them what you think they want to hear. Facing your grief must make room for emotional honesty with yourself and others. Without maintaining emotional honesty, your emotions can get out of control as the aggression leaks out from suppressing your feelings. You may even surprise yourself. Also, your attitude can put a strain on your relationships with loved ones who can get confused about your behavior.

Healing is in the owning that this is actually happening and living in the present moment with the desire to get through it one day at a time. Jeneel lost his daughter two years ago and shared that he was stuck in this space; moving on was difficult, and he did not realize he was hurting himself and his son, who needed him to continue living for both of them. His grief was blinding, and he forgot that his other child, whom he loved just as much as the child who died, needed his full attention as a person, as a parent, and as someone capable of being vulnerable. It is alright to allow family and friends to see us as humans, capable of hurting, while we are striving towards healing from the hurt.

Remember: you do not have to remain in the beginning stages of grief. Move through the cycle in the order that comes naturally to you. Most importantly, you do not want to be consumed by the memories of the past. Individuals who are overwhelmed by grief can have complications in healing, and subsequently, impacts their daily lives negatively. Those affected by your grief include dependent relatives, especially children and the elderly, who may grieve by extension as they watch your sadness spiral. Also, they may feel guilty about choosing to be happy in your presence and decide to take on the responsibility of being the caregiver even if they are not sure if they possess the skills to take care of you. Let them help you, but do not hand over the entire portfolio of your grief to those who love you. They may share in the grieving over the same loss, but do not allow them to grieve for losing you as well even though you are right there, visible, but not present. That is detrimental to any person.

It takes lots of courage to face grief when it looks like a vicious giant that you cannot slay. The good news is that God can slay this grief-giant for you. Have you heard of the giant slayer named Jesus? He has unlimited resources to leverage against grief and free you from its cruel grasp. Just call out to Jesus in faith believing that He is able to deliver you, and He will. "Lord help me" may seem like a small thing to say, but it is powerful when the person you're asking for help is omnipotent. Jerimiah 32:27 states, "I am the LORD, the God of all people. Is there anything too hard for Me to do?" Those are God's words, and He cannot lie. Trust Him and try Him!

Grieving can deplete all our energies, so looking to ourselves alone for the strength to win might give us a false sense of hope. Look beyond self. Sure, it's intimidating, but the truth is that we have access to the strength and courage necessary to slay the giant. However, we must be aware of our strengths and weaknesses; it is a trait of winners. When you're honest about your shortcomings, then you can begin to embrace solutions. Remember, our Bible text stated that "God gives us the Spirit of power..." This power includes physical strength, mental strength, emotional strength, and spiritual strength to win the battle over grief. We must, however, look to God, the ultimate source of power outside of ourselves. He is willing and able to pour out His sustaining power into our being to mobilize us with the desire to live an abundantly healthy life.

Now, ask yourself if you're having an issue with accepting grief as a part of your life. Do you think it makes you seem weaker to allow yourself to grieve properly? Do the feelings seem too impossible to consider? Then here are some helpful ways.

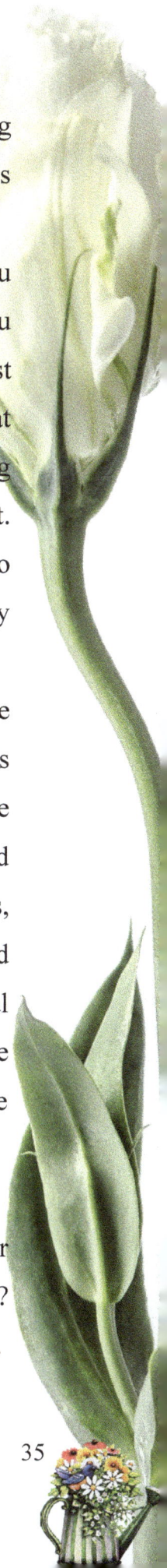

How to Step Out of Grief and Bloom: A Practical Guide By: Diana Rowe

The first step is to be honest with yourself despite feelings of fear, anger, or uncertainty. It's alright to be afraid of this new way that seems empty. But remind yourself that fear, though it is a human reaction, it is not a Godly response that speaks to how you should spend the rest of your life. In place of your human feeling of fear, "God gave you His Spirit of power." Take it. Also, it is fine to be angry and to want to hide from your grief. But do not hide. Even in times of anger, God understands. The sufficiency of His grace accommodates our authentic emotional response to death, divorce or other losses. God is not punitive amid our anger. But instead, He encourages and strengthens us to work towards understanding where we are right now; He wants us to use every minute on the clock to take one positive deep breath of reassurance that we are not alone or abandoned by Him. God says, "I will not leave you without the presence of My comfort in your time of bereavement; I will come to you." John 14:18.

Another step is to admit that you are negatively affected by your loss. That will enable you to look at yourself with kindness and patience. Other people may think you're taking too long to get over your grief; some may even tell you that it's time to move on. But do not let anyone rush your healing. When you get a cut on your finger, you do not criticize it and ask why it doesn't hurry up and heal; what is happening to your heart is more profound than a cut on your finger and needs a nurturing, gentle touch of encouragement, prayer, and support. Record your thoughts in your journal daily, confide in a trusted friend or relative, and listen to soothing Christian music that lifts your spirit. Reading and meditating on the promises of God found in the Bible is also great medicine for the healing of the mind. Isaiah 41:10 "Do not fear, for I am with you; Do not become anxious, for I am your God; I will strengthen you, surely, I will help you; surely, I will uphold you with My righteous right hand."

How to Step Out of Grief and Bloom: A Practical Guide By: Diana Rowe

Coping with the devastating effects of your loss is a necessary part of your journey. Do not let anyone invalidate your emotions. It is a step toward healing, no matter how long or difficult it is to take that first step. And you are strong and courageous enough to begin to take control of your life. Just believe Philippians 4:13 that says, "I can do all things through Jesus who strengthens me." Here, you have the beloved of heaven at the level of your faith to believe and ask for His help; He is ready and willing to be your strength in your weakest moment.

Life, as you once knew it, has changed, and you need to permit yourself to process these changes so that you can begin to adjust while you heal. You do not want to reside in a constant state of imbalance. All of us are naturally inclined to experience the various symptoms of grief. Don't be tempted to repress them to avoid adjusting to the radical changes that have shocked your life. This can bring on a whole variety of issues, from inexplicable and seemingly irrational fears, to anxiety or depressive disorders that can influence a negative pattern of behaviors. When this happens, many people turn to substance abuse to try to numb their pain, which can easily lead to addictions that take over their lives. It's very dangerous to deny or ignore that things have changed, and you're devastated at the prospect of dealing with everything alone, but remember, you are not alone. There is help for those who seek it. Psalm 46:1 reminds us that "God is our refuge and strength; He is a very present help in times of trouble." You may not look at grieving as being in trouble. Still, it is a form of trouble in your mind that disrupts equilibrium, and God wants you to know that He is there with you, and He also provides resources that can help you, including human pastoral counsel, a chaplain, clinicians, friends, and family.

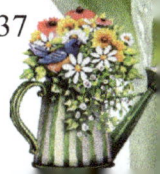

37

Chapter 6: Creating Moments While Grieving

Plants can create a positive impact even if they're growing in unfavorable conditions. The beautiful Lenten rose blooms in drought, heat, or cold all while in very poor soil.
You can bloom no matter what circumstances you might currently be in. Take time to be present and create beautiful moments; this will add enriching nutrients to your heart and help you to bloom.

The reality of change. Something that you used to rely on as a constant in your life is no longer there. It has now become a variable that may never be part of your life again, except in the ways that you still have control over, such as through prayers or to honor the memories of those you lost. There are many methods for dealing with death and loss, but they might all seem to pale in comparison to having the actual person or relationship back in your life. Nevertheless, you can carry on as you intentionally create new moments that count in a significant way.

Are you grieving a loss of security that you once had? Do you feel that you can never trust anything or anyone to remain in a familiar pattern? Are you feeling threatened by a projected tragedy or loss of some kind? Sometimes one loss can cause you to question everything else around you. It can shake your confidence in what used to be predictable and make you feel that the control you had over certain situations is now restricted or taken away. These feelings are not uncommon, which makes the grieving process even more crucial for your daily living to move beyond grief.

Before creating moments, it is essential to put things into perspective by admitting to yourself that (1) something devastating happened to me; (2) life will be different going forward; (3) I do not like what happened, and it is heart-breaking to accept it; (4) I am willing to take the painful steps to wholeness, although change is not easy, it is both necessary and possible.

As you grapple with the implications of your loss, you can take action to ease the transition. You can write letters to your loved one about the things you wanted to do or say but did not. There are specific pages in the companion journal to write your letter. This exercise will help to provide closure as you transfer your thoughts

38

and feelings into written and spoken words. Although you cannot give the person the letter physically, the act is not about the person you lost receiving a letter; it is about you opening the stress-vault of your heart so that the pressure from your thoughts is released. This outflow of your thoughts and emotions can help to alleviate some of your internal stress.

Participating in the planning of memorials can help to bring about closure while gaining the support of other people. The plan can include sharing with individuals from near and far with the use of social media that allows people to share their encouragement. Church or religious affiliations can also be a source of emotional and spiritual support during this time. Additionally, you can focus some of your energies on foundations that were dear to the heart of your loved one. For example, if your loved one walked for the cure for heart disease or diabetes, you can continue to make contributions to these organizations by participating in the walks, making financial donations, or volunteering to help those who are facing health challenges in these areas. Also, you can start a scholarship fund in memory of your loved one for students in medical schools or those wanting to attend or hospitals and other places that specialize in working towards a cure.

When the crowd is gone, the activities paused, you must prepare for the flood of memories as an ongoing part of your life. Hey, this is not a strange thing; if this never happens, that will be strange. In the same way, you can easily think of someone when they are alive, likewise, your thoughts of a person can surface after they die; your mind does not remove them as if they never existed. Life does not make room for us to run ahead of all our memories and squeeze them into submission, block them, or tie them together in a neat little pile and put them away. As we continue to live through grief, our love for those who are no longer with us remains in our hearts. Please note that we may have memorials and services to mark the loss and honor our loved ones, but we still carry the emotions and feelings we had before.

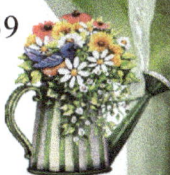

39

Therefore, we can expect that there will be a flood of emotions when birthdays, anniversaries, and holidays come around. In anticipation of these events, we can do something meaningful and healing such as celebrating those who were born on that date; honor a senior for services done the year your loved one was born; wear your loved one's favorite color to bring holiday cheer to a family in need; purchase some of your loved one's favorite things to give away. All these will help you to pass the time in a way that champions love and inspire others to live selflessly and intentionally while grieving. Grieving is part of living and that includes choosing to do good for the benefit of others. There's a direct blessing for your heart and mind when you purpose in your heart to live beyond your feelings and seek to uplift others who are in need.

You don't have to do it all alone. Remember, your family members and friends are not privy to your thoughts and feelings, don't forget to include them; let them know where you are emotionally and mentally. Help them to help you. They want to honor your feelings and the memory of your loved ones during these seasons; so, you can share ideas and let them help with the execution of the plans.

What else can you do? You can write some of the positive words that your loved one spoke to you when they were alive and keep them in your encouragement folder. I still remember positive quotes, silly moments, and joyful events with my late father and my sister. Sometimes I just break out in laughter because of the way they shared certain information with lots of humor. Facing your grief is not about immersing yourself in total sadness; remember, your loved ones' life had joy and happiness, fun and laughter too. Search your memory for some of those and bring in a resurgence of cheer that may start with a little smile and then the loudest laugh. Your loved one would want you to smile now and then. Permit yourself to SMILE A WHILE.

40

Don't forget that some of your family members and friends may have memories too. Give them permission to share their positive memories instead of making them feel as if they are insensitive if they mentioned a joyful time. The people around you may be missing the person you are grieving to some degree or other. Don't dismiss their feelings of wanting to bond with you in reminiscing, crying, or laughing. Don't try to manage their feelings or their memories; allow yourself to listen to how your loved one made positive contributions to other people's lives. Doing this may even inspire you to intentionally carry on this legacy of positivity in honor of your loved one.

On the contrary, if you anticipate that an upcoming event might cause some emotional difficulty, don't keep it to yourself. Tell the people in your life so they can begin to give you the space and comfort that you need to maintain your balance. It's perfectly fine to be sad. Do not neglect the importance of self-care during these times; do what you need to feel comfortable whether in a small group, large gathering, or a walk by the lake.

Find the section for holidays/special days in the grief journal and record your plan to help you get through the holidays.

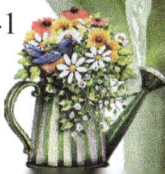

How to Step Out of Grief and Bloom: A Practical Guide By: Diana Rowe

Chapter 7: Processing Depression While Grieving

Many plants face harmful insects from time to time. Plant owners may see the problem but must also use the correct treatment so that the insects don't take over the entire plant. Sometimes the treatment can take several phases over a period of time, but the end goal is to have a healthy plant that blooms. So, at times you can experience depressive cycles but do not ignore them. Remember, you're on a path to bloom and you will succeed with the help of God and other resources.

Grief can warp our perspective, and depression can change it even further and convince us with false logic that we're worthless, and there's no hope (Mahali, Beshai, Feeney, & Mishra, 2020). Can I process depression when I am grieving? That is a question that many people ask. It is likely that the loss of your loved one brought on this depressive feeling.

Do a self-check:

Are you punishing yourself for having a positive outlook on life or for finding something positive that can come out of this loss? Do you have a change in your appetite, fatigue, loss of interest in daily activities (Zhang & Yen, 2015)? If your answer is yes, then you might be heading down the path of depression; this is not the short moment of feeling sad or hopeless when you first experienced the loss; this is more like entering into a permanent agreement with depression to become your default emotion. Don't sign this agreement! It is time to decide to reject signing your life away to depression! Your feelings may be out of balance, but that is not a perpetual state of mind. You will be made whole again by the power of God, your determination, and the help of caring people, and licensed counselors.

When people are grieving, it is often difficult for them to differentiate depression from grief:

Cadey was driving when she lost control of her car and hit a tree; which resulted in the death of her 10-year-old daughter. She spoke about her grief and tried to move on, but three and a half years later, she was drowning in the complications of her grief. We will learn more about this kind of complication in the next section.

42

Depression and grief are different; yet, at times, they seem so close that one who is grieving cannot tell them apart easily. That is true in Cadey's story. She had grief and depression all mixed up, but she was able to explain her feelings. She expressed the guilt she felt earlier in the grieving process, especially after she left the hospital. She thought perhaps after learning that something malfunctioned in her car, she would feel better, and for a while, she did. So, she assumed that after the funeral and trying to do right by the other children, the guilt would go away. But one day out of nowhere came this overwhelming feeling of guilt. This time she questioned everything about herself and her ability to do things right. She began isolating herself and making excuses to avoid family members, friends, and church. Then she could not look in the mirror anymore; she felt hatred towards herself and no longer wanted to drive the other children anywhere, for fear that she would crash and hurt them too.

Can you see Cadey here? From the outside looking in, do you recognize that those guilty feelings are completely irrational? Guess what? In Cadey's mind, her feelings make perfect sense; and her actions demonstrate her belief. Nevertheless, this is depression doing its finest work on the human brain. The fact is, Cadey is a strong, loving Christian mother of four beautiful children. She is stronger than what she is feeling. But she allowed the feelings to engulf her (partly to punish herself for surviving), and she didn't want to fight back because she accepted the depression contract and signed up to let depression become her new default emotion, at least for now.

Thank God that Cadey started learning about grief in the early portions of this course and found out that there is hope for her. As she learned about what was happening to her, she was able to look at the situation and see herself and used the companion journal to make step-by-step decisions to turn things around.

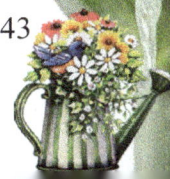

How to Step Out of Grief and Bloom: A Practical Guide By: Diana Rowe

Cadey followed the steps outlined in the companion journal that helped her to come out of isolation, take care of herself again, which helped her to take care of her children, forgive herself, and so much more. With the help of God, Cadey used the resources in the journal to fight against her emotional contract with depression. She is now continuing her journey to wellness.

Can you identify with Cadey? Then you too can overcome depression, introduced by your grief. Today, you can, like Cadey, begin to bloom again as the beautiful, strong, and resilient plant/flower you are! The same God who helped Cadey is more than able to help you!

Take a minute: record in your companion journal how you identify with Cadey. Write how you felt, why you were feeling that way, and what steps you took that was helpful or not helpful. What did you learn from this course that would be helpful in this situation?

Other symptoms of depression include preoccupation with your own death, feeling afraid to die, or wanting to die to escape depression. STOP! Don't sign this depression contract; it is not for you. God has a better plan for you, and He wants you alive to accomplish this plan.

Did you know that depression can cause some people to hallucinate? So, if you are hearing or seeing things that are not there, this is cause for concern, especially if you feel insecure or unhappy about your life in any way. STOP! Don't accept this depression contract; it is not for you. God wants you to know that you are "...remarkably and wondrously made..." (Psalm 139:14) in His image. He loves you, and He will bring you to equilibrium. Call on Jesus to stabilize your mind. Also, contact a pastoral counselor or another licensed counselor and share what is happening to you.

Are you having difficulty functioning at school, home, or work, especially after a loss? This can be unbelievably detrimental for your daily lifestyle; it truly

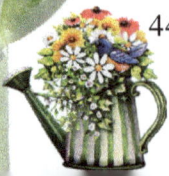

inhibits your progress to accomplish your short-term or long-term goals. As soon as you observe or sense the development of this pattern, just STOP! Don't accept this depression contract; it is not for you. 3 John 1:2 says, "Beloved, my prayer is for you to prosper in every way and be in good health physically, just as you are in good health spiritually." God made you to succeed in all the areas of life, and He will help you to prosper even in your health.

Slow movements exacerbate the difficulty in functioning, not keeping up the usual pace even around the house, at work, or school. Have you slowed down in an obvious way that you and those around you recognize (Zhang & Yen, 2015)? What has changed? After a loss, depression can zap your zeal to thrive and be productive as you did before. This can affect all aspects of our life and can worsen if you do not act quickly. So, examine yourself for this symptom. Then STOP! Don't accept this depression contract; don't sign it either; it is not for you. Remember: "The Sovereign LORD is my strength; He makes my feet like the feet of a deer, He enables me to tread on the heights…" Habakkuk 3:19. Do you see that God will strengthen you and give you swiftness of pace and the power to move about without the hindrance of slowness? That is an excellent consolation from God to you so that you can climb to lofty heights in your daily life. Oh yes, "I can do All things through Jesus who strengthens me." Philippians 4:13. Ask Jesus for the strength you need today. Go ahead, ask Him right now.

CAUTION: depression is not a joke. While it is not uncommon to experience it briefly during the stages of grief, it is not normal to continue in a depressed state, moving from a month to years. The best thing is to recognize the symptoms before they take over and paralyze your entire life. Don't self-medicate or use pills, alcohol, and other drugs to destroy yourself. Don't binge on anything, including food, to heal you mentally or emotionally. God will see you through this. Don't be ashamed to seek and accept appropriate help. Seek the Lord's help, seek the support of family,

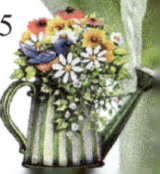

trusted friends, and the help of a licensed counselor. God wants you to be in balanced health; He loves you too much to want you to remain in a life-long state of sorrow.

Good news: You can incorporate some practical activities into your daily routine to help while dealing with depression. We all know the benefits of exercise; it can enhance our mood by releasing endorphins to combat stress and pain, and neurotransmitters like serotonin to fight depression and anxiety (Mikkelson et al., 2017). Exercise also helps with memory, retention (Mikkelson et al., 2017), and heart health (Hegberg et al., 2019). So, start by walking from one room to another until you can make it outside to get some fresh air and sunshine. Just start with five minutes and keep adding another five minutes every time. That can make a huge difference in your healing.

It's time to assess your list of things you like to do. Check your companion journal for some tips. In the meantime, if you like art, take a trip to the museum for some inspiration. How about serving at a local children's center? You may want to volunteer at the local food or soup kitchen. If you love animals, you may want to work at an animal shelter or adopt a pet. In fact, you can start a group with family and friends and the whole group can arrange to support a pet. Also, the group can start a fund for people in need of necessary supplies. There's also the opportunity to share the love of God to console someone who may be going through a tough time, even if they did not suffer the loss of a loved one. Start a Facebook group for people who have experienced your specific loss in your area or beyond and talk about ways you can help each other. Perhaps meet once per week or month (on the phone or online works too), and each person can bring a dish to share (you can share virtually if you cannot meet in person). That way, you can trade recipes and talk about cooking secrets. Make it fun and keep it light. That can certainly lift your mood, help you to come out of isolation, and participate in the joy and blessing of serving others.

How to Step Out of Grief and Bloom: A Practical Guide By: Diana Rowe

Chapter 8: Recognizing Complicated Grief

It is always good to recognize the weeds that can destroy a plant. Sometimes dangerous weeds can get so entangled with a plant that if you try to pluck it out without being careful to see what you're uprooting you can destroy the plant. Check for complicated grief and seek help to uproot this horrible weed; do not allow it to block your potential to bloom.

As you have probably noted from the previous section, normal grief can quickly turn complicated. Complicated grief is a condition that some people find themselves in, often without knowing that they are there. A deep feeling of sorrow characterizes this type of grief and completely consumes people's lives, rendering them hopeless. Many people go through the cycles of grief over and over without ever arriving at acceptance, which is an indication that they may be experiencing complicated grief.

Although depression is one of the main phases of grief, if left unmanaged, it can quickly spiral out of control and alter life as we know it. According to researchers, complicated grief lasts over a more extended time. People who find it hard to adjust to their new life without their loved ones, and are preoccupied with their loss, are suffering from complicated grief (Szuhany, Young, Mauro, García de la Garza, Spandorfer, Lubin, & Zisook, 2020).

We will explore how you can recognize complicated grief:

Complicated grief makes it challenging to end mourning. It can consume your life and keep you in the grief cycles with no desire to accept what happened (Szuhany, Young, Mauro, García de la Garza, Spandorfer, Lubin, & Zisook, 2020). That is extremely disruptive to the healing process.

Is your loss replaying in your mind every moment as if it just happened? Are your relationships with family and friends becoming more and more invisible while you stay focused on the loss itself? Are you unable to accomplish the simple goals for your daily living? Is there a longing in your heart that leads you to vehemently look in familiar places hoping to find the person you lost? Are you feeling confused

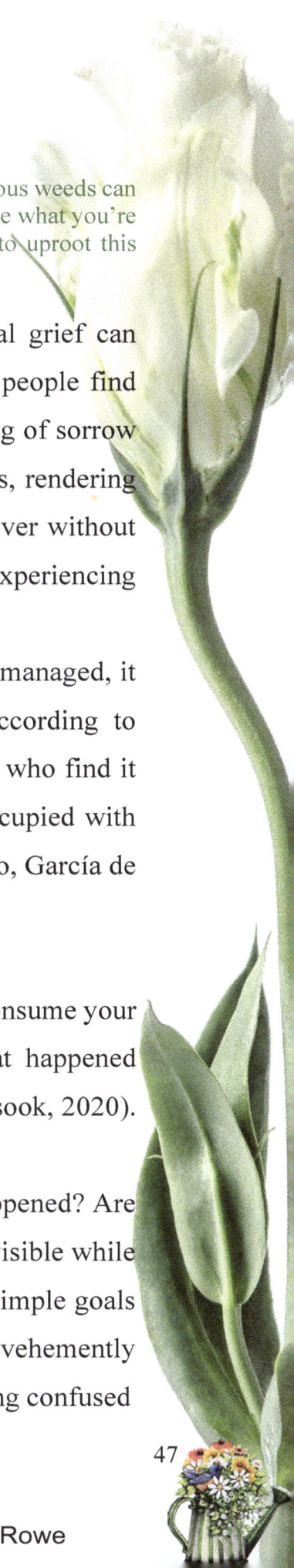

or disoriented about the events of the loss, trying to understand whether the loss occurred? Is your sadness deep and abiding, to the point that you reject all encouragement or cheer? So many people choose to take comfort in their imagination. How? They keep the person they lost alive and well in their imagination and function as if the person is still alive. Others battling complicated grief can experience a continuous sense of disbelief that can put a strain on their relationships with others who try to convince them of the reality (Shear, Simon, Wall, Zisook, Neimeyer, Duan, Reynolds, Lebowitz, Sung, Ghesquiere, Gorscak, Clayton, Ito, Nakajima, Konishi, Melhem, Meert, Schiff, O'Connor, First, Keshaviah, 2011).

Complicated grief has multiple layers and is more extreme than normal grief. Complicated grief includes a combination of long-term depression, anxiety, sleep disturbances, difficulty managing daily living, substance abuse, self-blame, shame, and wishing to die (Shear et al., 2011). Complicated grief involves rage and bitterness about the loss; the one who is grieving is furious at the person for leaving them, whether through death or even divorce; they can also be angry at anyone who reminds them of the loss (Shear et al., 2011). Not managing anger can cause irreparable damage to the relationships between family and friends. Long-term depression is also a part of complicated grief; it can leave a person to believe that without their loved one, life is meaningless. Are you feeling empty and angry? This emptiness and anger can foster the need to go to extreme measures to erase any trace of the person's existence without realizing it (Shear et al., 2011). That is not helpful for your healing or respecting the memory of your loved one. If you are divorced, blocking the person's existence in your mind does not help. The truth is, the person still exists, painful as it feels. You cannot avoid the pain of loss or the memories that naturally surface while grieving, even though it may be unbearable. At some point, reminders will confront you; so, it is best to face your loss using the resources that are available in this course, in the companion journal,

48

and other professional help as needed. In the case of divorce, you can still reorganize your life without that person. How? By narrowing your views to what is presently important and favorable for your growth. Also, remind yourself that you are fighting for yourself now, and full resuscitation is necessary because you have a 100% chance of surviving. Yes, you can make it!

Have you ever been told to get over your grief quickly? Perhaps being emotionally fragile is not something that family and friends can cope with, but you should not let this force you to act the way they want you to; that can make everything more complicated for you. Be in the moment and go through your experience naturally.

REMEMBER: Healthily dealing with your grief can help you to avoid complicated grief. Ask God for the strength to face the loss; also, do a self-check to determine if your symptoms are related to complicated grief. Now, use the checklist in your companion journal and make sure to inform your family members or close friends about what you are experiencing and your need for professional help to work through this intense grief.

Surviving a tragedy takes a toll on the whole person. However, this process is not a wasted trial; it is building up your resolve and bolstering your internal survival mechanism for every other situation. During this complicated grief, you will find that God is close to you, and your grief touches His heart. He will give you victorious strength in this battle! You will win!

Take a moment to record your feelings in your grief journal.

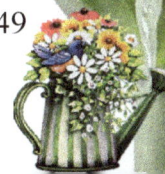

How to Step Out of Grief and Bloom: A Practical Guide By: Diana Rowe

Chapter 9: Patience and Forgiveness

Imagine planting your favorite flower in a pot and forgetting to add water. Even when it doesn't receive all the nutrients at the appointed time each day, the plant does not give up or complain; it patiently fights on. How about you? Are you quick to forgive yourself and be patient with yourself? It is a very tender regard that will nurture you to bloom at the right time.

In times of mourning, people quickly forget patience and forgiveness towards themselves. They may assume that it is selfish to regard themselves as needing patience and forgiveness. Some people believe that showing their emotions is weak or embarrassing, especially if they break down and cry publicly. They may find it awkward to allow others to see them vulnerable; this can cause some people to become impatient and upset that they are unable to keep it together. Remember that grieving is happening all around us; we never know what the person next door is going through. There are hundreds of people dealing with the symptoms of grief that you are experiencing at any given moment. Therefore, it is not uncommon for someone to understand that your emotions are out of balance during this painful time.

Healthy grieving can be raw and will need your undivided attention to process with patience. Thus, people are encouraged to take some time off from work or school to sort through their emotions in a reasonable time-frame. Do not be concerned if others do not understand why you need this time. It is imperative to take some time to yourself; you will need to take your time to look at what happened while exercising patience. Take the time to help yourself to move through your daily life one step at a time; use the suggestions in your companion journal to help you to organize your day. If you do not finish your tasks for that day, do not worry or get frustrated that it is taking too long. Let your body and mind go as far as you can, to do as much as you can, for that day. You can finish later. Be patient with you; it will help with your healing going forward.

As humans, we often try to connect events leading up to a tragedy, rather than accept that sometimes a tragedy stands alone. When we search our minds relentlessly, hoping for answers, and finding none, we can turn on ourselves. We can start to blame ourselves for what happened and how we could prevent it. We always want to change the outcome, but the reality is our proof, we simply cannot. Forgiveness is needed if we are not responsible and even if we are 100% responsible for what happened. Your loved one would not want you to go the rest of your life in a state of unforgiveness.

When Mr. Tomsien and his wife got sick from a virus, they did everything to get well; unfortunately, his wife died. Mr. Tomsien blamed himself and could not understand how the medicine worked for him and not for his wife. He felt terrible and thought that if he did not forgive himself, it was a well-deserved punishment. He soon learned that there was nothing he could do, and none of the events that led to his wife's death was his fault. As he walked through this course and the steps in the companion journal, he was able to move towards forgiving himself. The specific exercises about forgiveness in the journal helped significantly. It is not an easy process but is it possible.

Are you having a hard time forgiving yourself? Use the resources in the journal right now to start your journey towards forgiving yourself. You must learn to be alright with not being able to change the past and to forgive yourself for anything you may or may not have done wrong. The tragedy is awful, your pain is excruciating, but when someone else is facing a loss, you will be surprised at your level of compassion. While you are grieving, you do not realize that your tragedy can spark positive emotions inside your heart and give you greater insight for the future that allows you to help others.

Patience and forgiveness may not come easy when it is for ourselves, but it is necessary for our healing. The only power we have to make changes is to start to

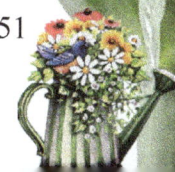

move forward because the past cannot change. It is always comforting to recognize that God knows all things. He knew when your loved one would die or leave your life through a divorce, and He knew exactly how you would react to the situation. Yet, in His Sovereign grace, He allowed everything to unfold. It is within the context of His grace that He wants you to forgive yourself as He has forgiven you for anything you may think is your fault. God has placed in you the capacity to endure tribulation without being consumed by it. Ask God to carry you; tell Him how you feel; pour out your heart to Him, and He will refresh you and breathe His restorative power in you so that you will desire to live with a deeper acceptance of being forgiven and free of guilt.

In addition to prayer, you can write in your journal about your feelings and daily experiences. Also, you can take some time to analyze which emotions are part of the grief stages so that with the help of God, you can more easily forgive yourself. Again, utilize the resources in your journal.

It is important to remember not to rush yourself in trying to face the future without forgiveness and patience. When it is tempting to question your ability to overcome, just remember that you can do this with the help of God and other resources. If you are thinking about giving up and not move forward, STOP! Take a deep breath and tell yourself, I am strong enough; I am not alone in this; I can, and I will make it to the other side, safely; I have a contribution to make in this life; someone needs my help out there, and I will serve in honor of my loved one. Or I will serve despite my divorce; my divorce may be the death of my relationship, but it is NOT the death of me.

REMEMBER: You have the power from the all-powerful God who stretched out the heavens and the earth; He is on your side. He will not send you to face the future and move forward alone; He will walk with you into the future as He promised in Deuteronomy 31:8 "The Lord Himself goes before you and will be with you; He will

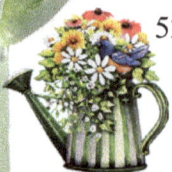

never leave you nor forsake you. Do not be afraid; do not be discouraged. Keep your hope in God; He will not fail you." In Psalm 32: 8, God promised that "I will instruct you and teach you in the way you should go; I will counsel you with My loving eye on you." This same God who created the universe and hung all the planets in perfect alignment loves you and will create peace and contentment out of the chaos of unforgiveness; He will align all your emotions in a balanced, healthy way and help you to forgive yourself. The freedom of forgiveness is all yours through Jesus, who paid the ultimate price for all kinds of forgiveness (towards other people and yourself).

Complete the activities regarding forgiveness in the grief journal.

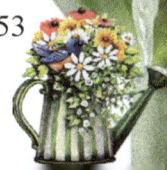

Chapter 10: New Perspective for Your New Normal

When you have a lovely plant, you try to find out what environment is best for it to flourish. If it needs very little sunlight and water twice per week you would never place it in the snow and add water daily. It is imperative for you to learn what it is that you need in your new environment to bloom. Perhaps learning a new hobby and taking some time to be grateful for everything in your life. At times we have to be transplanted to a new pot of soil (social, mental, emotional, spiritual, career or geographical location) to increase our chances to thrive. Place yourself in the best environment with the highest possibility to bloom. God will direct your path. Just ask Him to help.

When you are grieving, the future can look dreary with no positive aspiration in view. Missing our loved ones is normal, but don't forget that joy, peace, and happiness are still possible. The future is untouched, and it awaits you in a new and beautiful way; open your heart to endless opportunities.

Your dark time is fading behind one day at a time; leave it there; don't take it with you. You have a unique opportunity to spin your silver lining around the clouds in your many tomorrows. With the help of God, your friends, family, and other available resources, you can walk towards a new normal victoriously.

There is wisdom to gain from the losses we faced. As we reflect on the journey thus far, we can conclude that "life is short." Although we hear these words all the time, we sometimes apply them to the little time we had with our loved ones and hoped that we had more time with them; but, what if we take a different view of those words in terms of our next steps?

1. Since life is indeed short, then it is of utmost importance that you view every single day as a gift from God to improve your life and the lives of others around you. What do you do when someone gives you a gift that is unlike any other? You cherish it, right? Yes, your tomorrow is a brand-new day with brand new love, mercy, joy, and growth from God to you. Show your gratitude for the gift of a new day by using the valuable time given to create or participate in something that will make a positive contribution to your community.

2. Celebrate life at the time you are living it, or you may squander it.

How to Step Out of Grief and Bloom: A Practical Guide By: Diana Rowe

3. Allow your new normal always to include the big picture that can inspire you to greatness; something tragic can change your life negatively, but you can use the same tragedy to transform society positively.

4. Make all your relationships count. Let your family and friends know how deeply you care. Let the strangers know that they matter, too; do something for your local organizations to demonstrate your commitment to the development of the lives around you.

5. Examine the way you communicate with others and find ways to improve; make sure each person in your presence knows that they are valued.

6. Wear your badge of compassion daily and be grateful for the kindness that others showed to you in your time of need.

7. See your companion journal for additional suggestions that can help you on the new journey ahead.

By allowing yourself to lean on the power of God to take your mind out of the dark fog, you will realize there are things of value to learn from your experiences. A great lesson to learn is that there are different seasons in life that will challenge you to embrace the unknown with total trust in God. Remember, there is hidden value in every experience. Thus, there is a specific purpose for your life, and you can ask God to guide you to do what will be of most significant benefit to others. Every affirmative action taken is a step that helps to move you out of the grieving process and closer to healing.

Understanding death in a practical sense opens the mind for a healthy journey ahead. We know that the cycle of life includes being born and dying at some point. So, regardless who we choose to love, the material wealth we gain, the academic achievements and honors bestowed upon us, we must know who we are in relationship to all the things and people we care about. God has granted us the privilege to settle in our minds that we are going to stand, even if we must stand

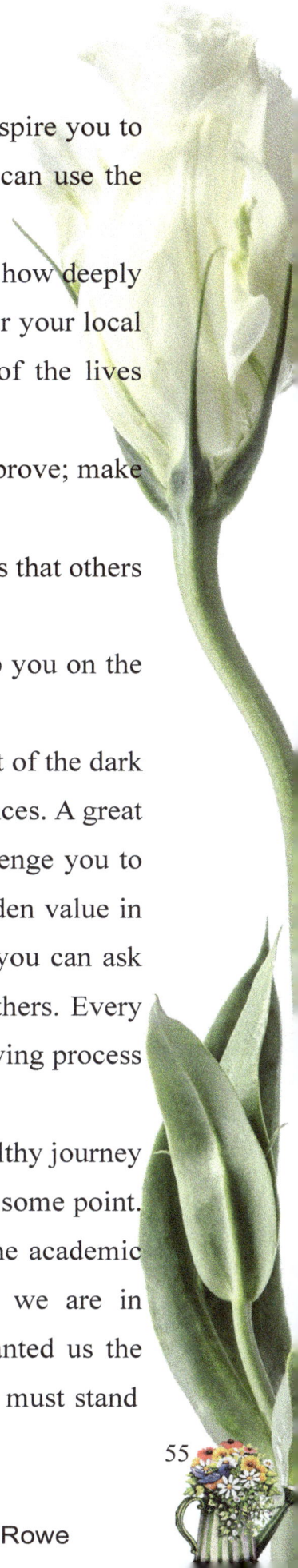

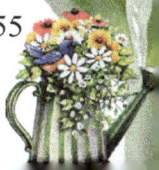

alone with no family, friends, or earthly possessions in the middle of a desert. Grief has the potential to push us to make a decision about who we are, who we are going to be, or how we will stand. You can, however, take the time to look at yourself, at the core of your being, and be devoted to who God says you are in Jesus: "…you are a joint-heir with Jesus." Romans 8:17. "…you are more than a conqueror through Jesus who loves you." Romans 8:37. Accept the attitude of a confident victor! Let this knowledge propel you to move forward no matter what.

A man by the name of Job served God yet, he lost all his earthly possessions, and all his children died in one day. Amid his pain and grief, Job was able to conclude this about God, "I know that You/God can do all things; no purpose of Yours can be thwarted." Job 42:2. Perhaps when one is alone with God, it is made clear that the loss of your loved ones happened under the Sovereign inscrutable wisdom of God, and your surrendering to His omniscience will allow Him to use your life for a purpose unknown to you. It is not easy to comprehend, that though God allowed a loss, it was never to cause you harm. Listen to these words spoken by God, "For I know the plans I have for you; I have plans to bless you and not to harm you, plans to give you hope and a future." Jeremiah 29:11.

God's purpose for your life is on His calendar despite your loss. Your loss and your thoughts about your loss cannot stop God's purpose.

So, celebrate life and living; it is the final step in coming out of grief and bloom!

Final Thoughts

As you strive for closure after a loss, with the help of God and other resources, you can declare victory over grief. You are highly loved by God who wants you to have abundant joy. God is not only there as your champion to coach you, but He wants you to know "your help comes from the Lord…" Psalm 121:2. God's help includes placing the right people to form a strong supportive network in your hour of need. Don't forget that it is alright to seek the help of a qualified professional who can assist with complicated grief. Your part includes accepting help, giving yourself the time, and patience you need to fully process your emotions, and accept this opportunity to enrich your life in a unique way you might never think possible.

This course and the companion journal were designed to give you some tools, shift your perspective to understand the grieving process, and help you to overcome grief and bloom in the summer breeze of life.

REMEMBER: You have an omnipotent, omniscient, omnipresent God whose compassion has no bounds to restore your broken pieces and make you whole again. You only need to call His name. He said, "Before you call me, I will answer; while you are still speaking, I will hear you." Isaiah 65:24. These words brought consolation to my own heart when I mourned my father's death. When I first heard the news, the God who sees and knows all things poured this beautiful promise all over my heart and answered me while I was calling His name to help me. He will do the same for you. "God's promise to all who mourn… is to give you the lasting beauty of His grace and presence, instead of the ashes of sorrow; the oil of joy, instead of mourning, and a garment that desires to praise God, instead of a heart burdened with despair…." Isaiah 61:3.

Grief is a reasonable reaction to the loss of someone significant in our lives, but that does not mean it is the end of our living. **Grief is another experience, though painful, that can equip us on the journey to intentionally listen, look,**

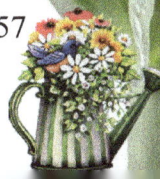

share, care and be sensitive to the needs of others and ourselves. It can help us to recognize the need to "give thanks in all circumstances…" 1Thessalonians 5:18. That may sound strange but thanking God for who He is will always be appropriate. Thanking God for what He is doing in your heart and for what He is going to do through your heart is really reassuring. God wants you to know that this experience is not a punishment but a moment that calls upon you to be a student of Sovereign grace.

Overcoming grief is possible because "…with God, all things are possible." Matthew 19:26.

Now that you've taken this course and start to use your journal, may God enable you with His power, His love, and a sound mind and body to continue your walk of victory today. Step Out of Grief! You Will Bloom!

Use your grief journal to write the steps for your goals as you bloom.

References:

Hegberg., N. J., Hayes, J. P. & Hayes, S. M. (2019). Exercise intervention in PTSD: A narrative review and rationale for implementation. Frontiers in Psychiatry, 10(133), 1-13. 19.

Holy Bible.

Kübler-Ross, Elisabeth. On Death and Dying. 1969. London: Routledge, 2009.

Mahali, S. C., Beshai, S., Feeney, J. R., & Mishra, S. (2020). Associations of negative cognitions, emotional regulation, and depression symptoms across four continents: International support for the cognitive model of depression. BMC psychiatry, 20(1), 18.

Mikkelson, K., Storjonavsky, L., Polenakovic, M., Bosevski, M., & Apostolopoulos, V. (2017). Exercise and mental health. Maturitas, 106, 48-56.

Shear, M. K., Simon, N., Wall, M., Zisook, S., Neimeyer, R., Duan, N., Reynolds, C., Lebowitz, B., Sung, S., Ghesquiere, A., Gorscak, B., Clayton, P., Ito, M., Nakajima, S., Konishi, T., Melhem, N., Meert, K., Schiff, M., O'Connor, M. F., First, M., … Keshaviah, A. (2011). Complicated grief and related bereavement issues for DSM-5. Depression and anxiety, 28(2), 103–117.

Shevchuk, N. A. (2008). Adapted cold shower as a potential treatment for depression. Medical hypotheses, 70(5), 995-1001.

Szuhany, K. L., Young, A., Mauro, C., García de la Garza, A., Spandorfer, J., Lubin, R., ... & Zisook, S. (2020). Impact of sleep on complicated grief severity and outcomes. Depression and anxiety, 37(1), 73-80.

Vingerhoets, A. (2013). Why only humans weep: Unravelling the mysteries of tears. Oxford University Press.

Zhang, J., & Yen, S. T. (2015). Physical activity, gender differences, and depressive symptoms. Health Services Research, 50(5), 1550-1573.

www.ingramcontent.com/pod-product-compliance
Lightning Source LLC
Chambersburg PA
CBHW042356030426
42336CB00030B/3499